BOWEL CANCER

Simple Suprising Secrect Of Understanding, Managing, Overcoming, Treatment And Recovery From Colorectal Cancer

Dr Ryan Jodan

INTRODUCTION

Definition and Overview

Colorectal cancer, often referred to as colon cancer or rectal cancer, is a type of cancer that starts in the colon or rectum. These are parts of the large intestine, which is the lower part of the digestive system. While the terms "colon cancer" and "rectal cancer" may refer to cancers in specific parts of the large intestine, they are often grouped together because of their similarities in terms of development, treatment, and risk factors.

Colorectal cancer is a significant health issue worldwide, ranking among the most common cancers in both men and women. It can affect individuals of any age, though it is more commonly diagnosed in older adults. The cancer typically begins as a small, benign growth known as a polyp, which can develop into cancer over time if left untreated.

The prevalence of colorectal cancer varies by region and population. Factors such as genetics, lifestyle, and diet play crucial roles in the risk of developing colorectal cancer. With advances in screening and early detection, the chances of successfully treating colorectal cancer have improved significantly. However, disparities in access to care and awareness can impact outcomes for different groups.

Purpose of the Book

This book aims to provide a comprehensive overview of colorectal cancer for a diverse audience, including patients, caregivers, medical professionals, and those seeking to better understand the disease. Whether you have recently been diagnosed, are supporting a loved one, or want to educate yourself about colorectal cancer, this book will offer valuable insights.

Here's what you can expect from this book:

- **In-Depth Information:** Detailed explanations of colorectal cancer, including its causes, symptoms, and progression, as well as the latest screening and diagnostic methods.

- **Treatment Options:** An exploration of the full range of treatment options, including surgical, non-surgical, and emerging therapies.

- **Living with Colorectal Cancer:** Practical advice and resources for patients and families coping with the disease, including strategies for managing side effects and maintaining quality of life.

- **Prevention and Risk Reduction:** Guidance on how to reduce your risk of colorectal cancer through lifestyle changes, diet, and screening.

- **Patient and Caregiver Stories:** Personal accounts from patients and caregivers to offer real-world perspectives on dealing with colorectal cancer.

- **Future Developments:** An overview of current research and advancements in the field of colorectal cancer.

This book strives to be an informative and supportive resource for anyone touched by colorectal cancer. By increasing understanding and awareness, the goal is to empower readers to make informed decisions about prevention, screening, treatment, and survivorship. Through this journey, we hope to contribute to better outcomes and improved quality of life for those facing colorectal cancer.

CHAPTER ONE

Basics of Colorectal Cancer

Anatomy and Physiology

The colon and rectum are essential parts of the digestive system, known collectively as the large intestine. The colon, also called the large bowel, is a muscular tube about 5 to 6 feet long that connects the small intestine to the rectum. It has four main sections: the ascending colon, transverse colon, descending colon, and sigmoid colon. The colon's primary function is to absorb water and nutrients from digested food and form solid waste, which is then stored in the rectum.

The rectum is the final section of the large intestine, measuring about 6 inches long. It serves as a temporary storage site for fecal matter before it is expelled from the body through the anus. The rectum is made up of different layers, including the mucosa, submucosa, and muscularis layers, which are important in understanding the progression of colorectal cancer.

What is Colorectal Cancer?

Colorectal cancer develops when cells in the lining of the colon or rectum begin to grow uncontrollably. This uncontrolled growth typically starts as a polyp, which is a small, benign (non-cancerous) growth. Over time, some polyps can change and become cancerous.

Cancer can develop in any part of the colon or rectum, and it can spread to other parts of the body if not detected and treated early. The progression of colorectal cancer can be classified into stages, ranging from stage 0 (where cancer is only in the innermost lining) to stage IV (where cancer has spread to other organs).

Risk Factors

Several factors can increase a person's risk of developing colorectal cancer:

- **Age:** The risk increases with age, particularly after age 50.

- **Family History and Genetics:** Individuals with a family history of colorectal cancer or certain inherited genetic conditions, such as Lynch syndrome and familial adenomatous polyposis (FAP), are at higher risk.

- **Lifestyle Factors:** Diets high in red and processed meats, low in fiber, and lack of physical activity are linked to higher risk.

- **Smoking and Alcohol Use:** Both smoking and heavy alcohol consumption are associated with an increased risk of colorectal cancer.

- **Obesity:** Excess body weight, particularly around the waist, can increase the risk.

- **Personal Medical History:** Those who have had colorectal polyps, inflammatory bowel disease, or other cancers may have a higher risk.

Symptoms and Early Detection

Colorectal cancer may not cause noticeable symptoms in its early stages, making screening crucial for early detection. However, as the disease progresses, the following symptoms may appear:

- **Changes in Bowel Habits:** Persistent diarrhea, constipation, or a change in stool consistency.

- **Rectal Bleeding or Blood in Stool:** Blood in or on the stool may appear bright red or dark.

- **Persistent Abdominal Discomfort:** Cramps, gas, bloating, or pain.

- **Unexplained Weight Loss:** Weight loss without a clear reason.

- **Fatigue and Weakness:** Feeling unusually tired or weak.

Early detection is key to successfully treating colorectal cancer. Regular screening, including colonoscopies and stool tests, can identify polyps or cancer early when they are most treatable. Recommendations for screening vary depending on individual risk factors, but many health organizations advise starting regular screening around age 45 to 50. Always consult with a healthcare provider for personalized screening recommendations.

Screening and Diagnosis

Screening Methods

Screening for colorectal cancer is crucial for detecting the disease early, often before symptoms appear. Early detection can lead to more effective treatment and better outcomes. Common screening methods include:

- **Colonoscopy:** A colonoscopy is the most comprehensive screening method. A flexible tube with a camera (colonoscope) is inserted through the rectum to examine the entire colon and rectum for polyps, abnormal growths, or cancer. Polyps can often be removed during the procedure, potentially preventing cancer development.

- **Sigmoidoscopy:** A sigmoidoscopy uses a shorter scope (sigmoidoscope) to examine the lower part of the colon (the sigmoid colon) and the rectum. It's less comprehensive than a colonoscopy but can still detect polyps and early-stage cancers.

- **Stool Tests:** These tests examine stool samples for hidden blood or DNA markers associated with colorectal cancer. Common tests include the fecal immunochemical test (FIT) and the guaiac-based fecal occult blood test (gFOBT). Stool DNA tests, such as Cologuard, look for cancer-related DNA changes.

- **Imaging Tests:** Virtual colonoscopy (CT colonography) uses CT scans to create images of the colon and rectum. This non-invasive method can detect polyps and other abnormalities but may lead to a follow-up colonoscopy if findings are suspicious.

Guidelines and Recommendations

Screening guidelines vary depending on age, risk factors, and personal medical history. Most health organizations recommend the following general guidelines:

- **Starting Age:** Routine screening is often recommended to begin at age 45 or 50 for individuals at average risk. Those with a family history of colorectal cancer or other risk factors may need to start screening earlier.

- **Screening Intervals:** The frequency of screening depends on the method used:

    - Colonoscopy: Every 10 years if no polyps are found.

    - Sigmoidoscopy: Every 5 years, sometimes in combination with FIT every year.

    - Stool tests: Annually.

    - CT colonography: Every 5 years.

Always consult with a healthcare provider for personalized screening recommendations.

Diagnostic Procedures

If a screening test indicates the possibility of colorectal cancer, additional diagnostic procedures may be performed:

- **Biopsy:** A biopsy involves taking a tissue sample from the suspicious area during a colonoscopy. The sample is examined under a microscope to determine if it contains cancerous cells.

- **Imaging Techniques:** Additional imaging tests, such as CT scans, MRI scans, or PET scans, may be used to assess the extent of cancer and determine if it has spread to other areas of the body.

Understanding Staging

Staging is a critical part of diagnosing colorectal cancer and guides treatment decisions. The stages are determined by the extent of cancer's spread:

- **Stage 0:** Also known as carcinoma in situ, cancer is only in the innermost layer (mucosa) of the colon or rectum.

- **Stage I:** Cancer has grown through the mucosa and submucosa but not beyond the colon or rectum wall.

- **Stage II:** Cancer has grown into or through the muscularis layer of the colon or rectum but not yet spread to nearby lymph nodes.

- **Stage III:** Cancer has spread to nearby lymph nodes but not to other parts of the body.

- **Stage IV:** Cancer has spread to distant organs, such as the liver or lungs.

Staging is usually determined through a combination of imaging tests and biopsy results. Accurate staging helps inform the treatment plan and predict the patient's prognosis.

CHAPTER TWO

Treatment Options

Once colorectal cancer is diagnosed and staged, treatment options can be explored. Treatment plans depend on several factors including the cancer's stage, the tumor's location, the patient's overall health, and personal preferences. Here, we discuss surgical and non-surgical treatments, as well as emerging therapies and research.

Surgical Treatments

Surgery is the most common treatment for colorectal cancer, particularly when the cancer is localized and has not spread to distant parts of the body. Surgical options include:

- **Polypectomy and Local Excision:** These minimally invasive procedures remove polyps or small cancers in the early stages. During a colonoscopy, polyps can be removed (polypectomy), or small tumors can be excised (local excision).

- **Resection:** For cancers that have grown beyond the mucosa, the surgeon may perform a partial resection, removing the section of the colon or rectum with the cancer and a margin of healthy tissue. The remaining healthy ends of the colon or rectum are then reconnected (anastomosis).

- **Colectomy:** In some cases, part or all of the colon may need to be removed (colectomy). There are different types of colectomies, such as right, left, or total colectomy, depending on the location and extent of the cancer.

- **Colostomy or Ileostomy:** Sometimes, if an anastomosis is not possible or needs to heal, the surgeon may create a stoma (an opening in the abdominal wall) to divert waste into a bag. This can be temporary or permanent, depending on the circumstances.

- **Laparoscopic Surgery:** Also known as minimally invasive surgery, this approach uses smaller incisions and specialized instruments to remove the cancer. Recovery is typically faster than traditional open surgery.

Non-surgical Treatments

Non-surgical treatments are often used in combination with surgery or as primary treatments when surgery isn't an option. These include:

- **Chemotherapy:** Chemotherapy uses drugs to kill cancer cells. It may be used before surgery (neoadjuvant) to shrink tumors, after surgery (adjuvant) to reduce the risk of recurrence, or as the main treatment for advanced cancers.

- **Radiation Therapy:** Radiation therapy uses high-energy radiation to target and kill cancer cells. It's more commonly used for rectal cancer than colon cancer, often before surgery to shrink tumors or as palliative treatment in advanced cases.

- **Targeted Therapy:** Targeted therapy involves drugs that specifically attack cancer cells based on their genetic makeup or molecular changes. This type of therapy can be more precise and cause fewer side effects than traditional chemotherapy.

- **Immunotherapy:** Immunotherapy works by boosting the patient's immune system to recognize and fight cancer cells. It's primarily used in cases of advanced colorectal cancer with specific genetic markers.

Emerging Treatments and Research

Research in colorectal cancer is ongoing, and new treatments and technologies are constantly being developed. Some promising areas of research include:

- **Precision Medicine:** Personalized treatments based on a patient's genetic profile or the genetic characteristics of the cancer are being explored. This approach aims to target cancer more effectively while minimizing side effects.

- **New Drug Therapies:** Researchers are investigating novel drugs and drug combinations to improve outcomes for colorectal cancer patients.

- **Immunotherapy Advances:** Continued research in immunotherapy is leading to new strategies for harnessing the body's immune system to fight colorectal cancer more effectively.

- **Liquid Biopsies:** Liquid biopsies, which analyze blood samples for cancer markers, are being studied as a non-invasive method to monitor treatment response and detect recurrence.

- **Advances in Screening:** New screening methods, such as improved stool tests and breath tests, are being explored to increase early detection rates and improve patient outcomes.

These emerging treatments and areas of research hold promise for improving colorectal cancer management and outcomes. Keeping up with the latest advances can help patients and healthcare providers make informed decisions about the best course of action.

Living with Colorectal Cancer

A diagnosis of colorectal cancer can bring a range of emotions and challenges for patients and their families. Coping with the disease and its treatment requires a holistic approach that encompasses emotional support, managing side effects, and making beneficial lifestyle changes.

Coping Strategies

Living with colorectal cancer can be a difficult journey for both patients and their loved ones. Emotional and psychological support is essential to navigate this challenging time:

- **Open Communication:** Talking openly with family, friends, and healthcare providers can help patients express their feelings and concerns. It can also help loved ones understand what the patient is going through.

- **Support Groups:** Joining a support group can provide comfort and understanding from others who are going through similar experiences. These groups can offer valuable emotional support and practical advice.

- **Counseling and Therapy:** Professional counseling can help patients and families manage emotions such as anxiety, depression, and stress. Cognitive-behavioral therapy (CBT) and other therapeutic approaches can provide coping strategies.

- **Mindfulness and Relaxation Techniques:** Practices such as meditation, yoga, and deep breathing exercises can help reduce stress and improve mental well-being.

- **Creative Outlets:** Engaging in hobbies and creative activities can offer a sense of purpose and distraction from the challenges of cancer.

- **Spiritual Support:** For those with spiritual or religious beliefs, seeking guidance and comfort from faith-based communities or clergy can be helpful.

Managing Side Effects

Colorectal cancer treatment can cause a range of side effects, which vary depending on the type and duration of treatment. Addressing these side effects can improve quality of life:

- **Fatigue:** Fatigue is a common side effect of cancer and its treatments. Resting as needed and prioritizing activities can help manage fatigue.

- **Nausea and Vomiting:** Medications known as antiemetics can help control nausea and vomiting. Eating small, frequent meals and avoiding strong smells can also be beneficial.

- **Diarrhea or Constipation:** Depending on the treatment, patients may experience changes in bowel habits. Staying hydrated, adjusting dietary fiber intake, and consulting a healthcare provider for medication can help manage these issues.

- **Mouth Sores:** Chemotherapy and radiation can cause mouth sores. Using special mouthwashes and avoiding irritating foods can alleviate discomfort.

- **Skin Changes:** Radiation therapy can cause skin irritation or burns. Keeping the affected area clean and using recommended creams or ointments can help.

- **Peripheral Neuropathy:** Some chemotherapy drugs can cause nerve damage, leading to tingling, numbness, or pain in the extremities. Medications and physical therapy can help manage these symptoms.

Nutrition and Lifestyle

Maintaining a healthy lifestyle can support recovery and overall well-being during and after treatment:

- **Balanced Diet:** Eating a variety of fruits, vegetables, whole grains, and lean proteins provides essential nutrients for healing and recovery. Patients should follow their healthcare provider's recommendations regarding dietary changes.

- **Hydration:** Staying hydrated is crucial, especially when experiencing side effects like diarrhea or vomiting. Water, herbal teas, and clear broths are good options.

- **Exercise:** Light to moderate exercise, such as walking or gentle yoga, can boost energy levels, improve mood, and help maintain physical health. Consult a healthcare provider before starting any new exercise program.

- **Weight Management:** Maintaining a healthy weight can improve outcomes and reduce the risk of complications. Work with a healthcare provider or dietitian to develop a personalized plan.

- **Limiting Alcohol and Tobacco:** Reducing or eliminating alcohol and tobacco use can improve treatment outcomes and lower the risk of complications and recurrence.

Living with colorectal cancer requires a multifaceted approach that includes emotional, physical, and dietary support. By adopting coping strategies, managing side effects, and making healthy lifestyle choices, patients can enhance their quality of life during and after treatment.

CHAPTER THREE

Survivorship and Beyond

Survivorship is an important aspect of the colorectal cancer journey. Once treatment is completed, patients transition into a new phase where long-term monitoring and care are crucial. This chapter discusses survivorship care, understanding the risk of recurrence and secondary cancers, and strategies for maintaining a good quality of life post-treatment.

Survivorship Care

Survivorship care involves ongoing monitoring and support for individuals who have completed colorectal cancer treatment. This type of care is tailored to the unique needs of each survivor and includes:

- **Follow-Up Appointments:** Regular check-ups with healthcare providers to monitor health, discuss any new symptoms, and conduct routine screenings for recurrence.

- **Surveillance Tests:** Depending on the stage and type of cancer, follow-up colonoscopies, imaging scans, and blood tests may be recommended to check for recurrence.

- **Late Effects Monitoring:** Treatment for colorectal cancer can cause late effects such as cardiovascular issues, neuropathy, or bone density loss. Monitoring and managing these effects are important for long-term health.

- **Managing Comorbidities:** Survivors may have other chronic conditions such as diabetes or heart disease. Coordinated care with specialists can help manage these conditions alongside cancer survivorship.

- **Rehabilitation and Physical Therapy:** Depending on treatment and surgery, physical therapy or rehabilitation may be necessary to improve strength, mobility, and overall function.

Recurrence and Secondary Cancers

Understanding the risk of recurrence and secondary cancers is vital for survivors. Although not all survivors experience a recurrence, it's important to be aware of the potential risks:

- **Risk of Recurrence:** The risk of cancer returning varies depending on the initial stage, location, and other factors. Close monitoring and surveillance tests can help detect recurrence early.

- **Prevention of Recurrence:** Lifestyle changes such as maintaining a healthy diet, regular physical activity, and avoiding tobacco and excessive alcohol can help reduce the risk of recurrence.

- **Secondary Cancers:** Survivors may have an increased risk of developing secondary cancers, either in the colon or rectum or in other parts of the body. Regular screening and healthy lifestyle choices can help mitigate this risk.

Quality of Life

After completing treatment, many survivors focus on rebuilding their lives and maintaining a good quality of life. Strategies for doing so include:

- **Emotional and Mental Well-being:** Seeking counseling, therapy, or support groups can help survivors cope with the emotional impact of cancer and its treatment.

- **Social Support:** Maintaining connections with family and friends and participating in social activities can contribute to a positive outlook and better quality of life.

- **Healthy Lifestyle Choices:** Continuing to prioritize a balanced diet, regular exercise, and stress management techniques can support long-term health and well-being.

- **Career and Financial Concerns:** Survivors may face challenges returning to work or managing finances due to medical expenses. Seeking support from career counselors or financial advisors can help address these concerns.

- **Hobbies and Interests:** Pursuing hobbies and activities that bring joy and fulfillment can enhance quality of life and provide a sense of purpose.

- **Advocacy and Education:** Sharing experiences and raising awareness about colorectal cancer can empower survivors and provide a sense of satisfaction and community involvement.

Survivorship marks the beginning of a new chapter in the journey with colorectal cancer. Through regular monitoring, preventive measures, and lifestyle choices, survivors can maintain their health and well-being while finding fulfillment in post-treatment life.

Prevention and Risk Reduction

Colorectal cancer prevention and risk reduction focus on making lifestyle modifications, utilizing screening and surveillance, and understanding one's genetic risk. This chapter discusses these key areas and how they can help individuals maintain their health and lower their risk of developing colorectal cancer.

Lifestyle Modifications

Adopting healthy lifestyle habits is an essential component of colorectal cancer prevention. These modifications can significantly reduce risk and improve overall health:

- **Healthy Diet:** Consuming a diet rich in fruits, vegetables, whole grains, and legumes provides important nutrients and fiber. Limiting red and processed meats, as well as high-fat and high-sugar foods, can also lower colorectal cancer risk.

- **Regular Exercise:** Engaging in regular physical activity can help maintain a healthy weight and improve overall health. Aim for at least 150 minutes of moderate-intensity aerobic exercise or 75 minutes of vigorous-intensity exercise per week.

- **Weight Management:** Maintaining a healthy body weight is crucial for reducing colorectal cancer risk. This can be achieved through a balanced diet and regular exercise.

- **Avoiding Tobacco and Limiting Alcohol:** Smoking increases the risk of colorectal cancer, as well as many other cancers. Quitting smoking can lower this risk. Limiting alcohol consumption to moderate levels (up to one drink per day for women and up to two drinks per day for men) can also reduce risk.

Screening and Surveillance

Regular screening is one of the most effective ways to prevent colorectal cancer. Early detection allows for the identification and removal of precancerous polyps before they become cancerous, as well as the diagnosis of cancer in its earlier, more treatable stages:

- **Types of Screening:** Common screening methods include colonoscopy, sigmoidoscopy, and stool tests such as fecal immunochemical test (FIT) and stool DNA tests.

- **Screening Recommendations:** The age at which screening should begin varies depending on risk factors, but general guidelines recommend starting screening around age 45 or 50 for average-risk individuals. Those with higher risk, such as a family history of colorectal cancer, may need to begin screening earlier.

- **Screening Intervals:** The recommended frequency of screening depends on the method used:

- Colonoscopy: Every 10 years if no polyps are found.

  - Sigmoidoscopy: Every 5 years, sometimes in combination with FIT annually.

  - Stool tests: Annually.

- **Follow-Up and Surveillance:** Regular follow-up colonoscopies and other surveillance methods are important for individuals who have had polyps removed or been treated for colorectal cancer.

Genetic Counseling and Testing

Individuals with a family history of colorectal cancer or certain genetic conditions may benefit from genetic counseling and testing:

- **Family History:** A family history of colorectal cancer, particularly in close relatives or at a young age, may indicate a higher risk of the disease. Genetic counseling can help assess this risk.

- **Genetic Counseling:** A genetic counselor can review family history, assess risk, and discuss the potential benefits and risks of genetic testing. They can also offer guidance on preventive measures and screening protocols.

- **Genetic Testing:** Genetic testing can identify specific inherited conditions that increase colorectal cancer risk, such as Lynch syndrome and familial adenomatous polyposis (FAP). Knowing one's genetic risk can inform screening and prevention strategies.

- **Preventive Measures:** Those identified as having an increased genetic risk may consider more frequent screenings and other preventive measures, such as prophylactic surgery, in some cases.

By incorporating healthy lifestyle habits, adhering to recommended screening protocols, and understanding genetic risk, individuals can take proactive steps to prevent colorectal cancer or detect it early when treatment is most effective.

CHAPTER FOUR

The Future of Colorectal Cancer

The field of colorectal cancer is evolving rapidly as research progresses and new treatments emerge. In this chapter, we explore advancements in research and the growing importance of personalized medicine in the treatment of colorectal cancer.

Advancements in Research

Research in colorectal cancer is an active field, with scientists investigating new methods of prevention, detection, and treatment. Some current trends in research include:

- **Innovative Screening Methods:** Researchers are exploring new, non-invasive screening methods such as blood tests, breath tests, and advanced stool tests to improve early detection rates and patient compliance.

- **Novel Therapies:** Clinical trials are testing new drugs and treatment combinations, including novel chemotherapy agents, targeted therapies, and immunotherapies.

- **Immunotherapy Developments:** Immunotherapy continues to show promise in colorectal cancer treatment, especially for patients with certain genetic markers. Research is focusing on expanding the use of immunotherapy and improving its effectiveness.

- **Microbiome Research:** Studies on the gut microbiome (the community of microorganisms in the digestive tract) are providing insights into how the microbiome influences colorectal cancer development and treatment response. Researchers are exploring ways to manipulate the microbiome to prevent or treat colorectal cancer.

- **Precision Surgery and Radiation Therapy:** Advancements in surgical techniques, such as robotic-assisted surgery, and radiation therapy, such as stereotactic body radiation therapy (SBRT), are leading to more precise and effective treatments with fewer side effects.

Personalized Medicine

Personalized medicine, also known as precision medicine, tailors treatment to individual patients based on their genetic makeup, the genetic characteristics of their tumor, and other personal factors. This approach aims to maximize treatment effectiveness while minimizing side effects.

- **Genetic Profiling:** Genetic testing of tumors helps identify specific mutations that can be targeted with precise therapies. This allows for treatments that directly target cancer cells, sparing healthy tissues and reducing side effects.

- **Targeted Therapies:** Therapies that target specific genetic mutations in cancer cells can be more effective than traditional chemotherapy and may offer better outcomes for certain patients.

- **Immunotherapy:** Immunotherapy can be personalized by identifying which patients are likely to respond based on specific genetic markers, such as microsatellite instability-high (MSI-H) status or mismatch repair deficiency.

- **Pharmacogenomics:** Pharmacogenomics involves studying how a patient's genes affect their response to medications. This can help determine the most effective and safe drug combinations for each individual.

- **Predictive Biomarkers:** Researchers are exploring biomarkers that can predict treatment response, such as circulating tumor DNA (ctDNA), which can guide treatment decisions and monitor disease progression.

- **Tailored Screening Protocols:** Personalized risk assessment can lead to more individualized screening recommendations, based on factors such as genetic risk, family history, and lifestyle.

Personalized medicine is a promising direction in the future of colorectal cancer treatment. By leveraging genetic and molecular insights, healthcare providers can offer targeted and effective treatments tailored to each patient's unique profile. This approach has the potential to improve outcomes and quality of life for colorectal cancer patients. As research continues, we can expect even more significant advancements in the prevention, detection, and treatment of colorectal cancer.

Patient Stories and Perspectives

Personal experiences can provide valuable insight into the journey of living with colorectal cancer and the challenges and triumphs faced along the way. This chapter features stories from patients, survivors, and caregivers, highlighting their unique perspectives.

First-Hand Experiences

Hearing from patients and survivors offers a deeper understanding of the emotional, physical, and psychological aspects of dealing with colorectal cancer. These stories demonstrate resilience, courage, and the importance of community support.

- **Jane's Story:** Jane was diagnosed with stage II colon cancer at the age of 52. After undergoing surgery and chemotherapy, she experienced a rollercoaster of emotions. Jane found solace in support groups and leaned on her family for strength. She emphasizes the importance of listening to her body and trusting her medical team.

- **Mike's Journey:** Mike, a 65-year-old grandfather, discovered he had stage III rectal cancer during a routine colonoscopy. Despite initial fears, Mike approached his treatment with optimism and determination. He credits his positive outlook and the support of his wife for helping him navigate radiation, chemotherapy, and surgery.

- **Samantha's Experience:** Samantha, diagnosed with Lynch syndrome at age 40, was proactive in her approach to screening and surveillance. Her story highlights the importance of genetic counseling and early detection. Samantha's family history prompted her to advocate for regular screenings and preventive measures.

Caregiver Perspectives

Caregivers play a crucial role in supporting loved ones with colorectal cancer. Their stories reveal the emotional and practical challenges they face, as well as the rewards of being there for their loved ones.

- **Tom's Role as a Caregiver:** Tom's wife, Susan, was diagnosed with rectal cancer when she was 58. As her primary caregiver, Tom balanced his job with taking Susan to appointments and helping her manage side effects. His story underscores the importance of self-care for caregivers and the need for support networks.

- **Maria's Support for Her Father:** Maria's father, who had never missed a routine screening, was diagnosed with stage IV colon cancer at 70. Maria found it challenging to watch her father go through treatment, but she remained his constant companion. She emphasizes the importance of open communication and creating moments of joy during difficult times.

- **Samantha's Experience as a Daughter:** Samantha's mother was diagnosed with colorectal cancer at 63. As a daughter and caregiver, Samantha experienced mixed emotions, including fear, sadness, and hope. She found strength in their shared memories and used this experience to advocate for colorectal cancer awareness and prevention.

These stories from patients, survivors, and caregivers offer a glimpse into the reality of living with colorectal cancer. They demonstrate the importance of resilience, community support, and open communication in navigating the cancer journey. These perspectives can inspire and offer hope to others facing similar challenges.

36

CHAPTER FIVE

Conclusion

In conclusion, this book has provided a comprehensive overview of colorectal cancer, covering its definition, risk factors, diagnosis, treatment, survivorship, prevention, and the future of research and personalized medicine. Throughout the journey, we have also heard the first-hand experiences of patients, survivors, and caregivers, offering valuable insight into the human aspect of living with colorectal cancer.

Summary and Key Takeaways

Here are some of the most important points from the book:

- **Understanding Colorectal Cancer:** Colorectal cancer affects the colon and rectum, and early detection is key to successful treatment and survival. Awareness of risk factors and symptoms can prompt timely medical intervention.

- **Screening and Diagnosis:** Regular screening methods such as colonoscopy, sigmoidoscopy, and stool tests are essential for early detection. Surveillance and diagnostic procedures are crucial for confirming diagnoses and staging.

- **Treatment Options:** Treatment varies depending on the stage and location of the cancer. Surgical options, chemotherapy, radiation therapy, immunotherapy, and targeted therapies offer a range of approaches tailored to the patient's needs.

- **Living with Colorectal Cancer:** Coping strategies, managing treatment side effects, and making beneficial lifestyle changes are important aspects of living with colorectal cancer.

- **Survivorship and Beyond:** Long-term monitoring, addressing late effects of treatment, and taking preventive measures against recurrence and secondary cancers are key components of survivorship.

- **Prevention and Risk Reduction:** Adopting healthy lifestyle habits, adhering to screening protocols, and understanding genetic risk can help individuals prevent colorectal cancer or catch it early.

- **The Future of Colorectal Cancer:** Research advancements and personalized medicine offer hope for more effective treatments tailored to individual patients.

- **Patient Stories and Perspectives:** The experiences of patients, survivors, and caregivers offer insight into the emotional and practical aspects of dealing with colorectal cancer, emphasizing the importance of community support and resilience.

- **Colorectal Cancer Support Group:** Many hospitals and cancer centers offer support groups for those dealing with colorectal cancer. These groups provide emotional support and a sense of community.

This book aims to empower readers with knowledge about colorectal cancer and provide guidance on prevention, treatment, and survivorship. By staying informed and seeking support when needed, individuals can navigate the challenges of colorectal cancer and work toward better health and well-being.

www.ingramcontent.com/pod-product-compliance
Lightning Source LLC
Chambersburg PA
CBHW051858250726
48659CB00006B/2290